HYPOALLERGENIC DIET

FOR NOVICES

Enriched Recipes, Foods, Meal Plan & Procedures That Focuses On Discovering The Path To Better Health, Wellness And More

DR. MATEO GABRIEL

DISCLAIMER

The information in this book is only meant to be used for general reading. In any way, the author and publisher do not promise or represent that the information in this work is full, correct, reliable, appropriate, or available. This includes any warranties that are expressed or implied. Because of this, you should only rely on this material at your own risk.

This book is not meant to replace professional help. If you have any questions about a subject, you should always get help from a qualified expert. The author and distributor of this book are not responsible for how the information in it is used or abused.

The author's thoughts and feelings are shown in this book. They do not necessarily represent the official policy or stance of any other person, group, employer, or business.

Any third-party material that you can get to through this book is not endorsed or backed by the author or publisher.

The information in this book is correct at the time it was published, after all possible checks. However, the author and distributor are not responsible for any loss, damage, or inconvenience that may be caused by mistakes or omissions.

TABLE OF CONTENTS

CHAPTER ONE

INTRODUCTION TO HYPOALLERGENIC DIET

KNOWLEDGE OF HYPOALLERGENIC DIETS

As far as dietary habits go, the idea of hypoallergenic diets has become something that people who want to control and lessen food-related allergy reactions must take into account. A hypoallergenic diet offers a carefully chosen assortment of foods that are less likely to cause unfavorable immunological responses, with the main goal being to reduce the chance of causing allergic reactions. Comprehending the complexities of hypoallergenic diets entails exploring the fundamental characteristics of allergens, sensitivity, and the wider effects that dietary decisions can have on a person's general health.

A HYPOALLERGENIC DIET: WHAT IS IT?

Fundamentally, a hypoallergenic diet is a nutritional strategy designed to lessen the chance of allergic reactions to specific foods. This diet plan calls for cutting out or restricting foods that are frequently causing allergies, like dairy, gluten, nuts, and shellfish. The goal is to reduce food allergy symptoms, which can range from minor discomfort to severe and potentially fatal reactions. To guarantee a thorough and efficient approach to managing food-related sensitivities, working with healthcare specialists such as allergists and dietitians is often necessary when detecting allergens and creating a hypoallergenic diet.

THE VALUE OF EATING HYPOALLERGENIC FOODS

When one considers the potentially dire effects of allergy responses, the importance of eating hypoallergenically becomes clear. Food allergies and sensitivities can cause a variety of symptoms in its sufferers, such as respiratory troubles, skin disorders, gastrointestinal distress, and in severe situations, anaphylaxis. A hypoallergenic diet can help people reduce these risks and improve their quality of life in general. Furthermore, hypoallergenic diets are important for people who have previously been diagnosed with food allergies as well as for people who are more likely to experience allergic reactions in the future.

COMMON SENSITIVITIES AND ALLERGENS

It is essential to have a solid awareness of common allergies and sensitivities to fully understand the concepts behind hypoallergenic diets. Allergens that are most commonly encountered are gluten, dairy, nuts, eggs, soy, and shellfish, among others. These compounds may cause allergy reactions in those who are sensitive to them by inducing immunological responses. Understanding the variety of allergies enables the development of hypoallergenic diets with greater focus and efficacy. Furthermore, it's critical to recognize the difference between sensitivities and real allergies because it affects the level of dietary restriction required for an individual to maintain optimal health.

Learning about hypoallergenic diets entails a comprehensive investigation of allergies, sensitivity, and the critical function that these dietary decisions play in promoting well-being. Understanding the principles of hypoallergenic food empowers people to control their current allergies or lower their chance of experiencing negative reactions, which in turn promotes a healthier and more balanced way of living.

CHAPTER TWO

THE FUNDAMENTALS OF SENSITIVITIES AND ALLERGIES

AN OVERVIEW OF ALLERGIES

Reactions of the immune system to substances that are generally safe for most people result in allergies. The main job of the immune system is to protect the body from dangerous intruders like germs and viruses. Allergies, on the other hand, result from the immune system mistaking some substances—known as allergens—for dangers. This sets off an overreaction that releases several substances, including histamine, which aggravates allergy symptoms. Allergies can impact different body systems and organs in a variety of ways.

MANY ALLERGY TYPES

Allergies come in many different forms; however, they can be roughly divided into multiple groups according to the type of allergen and the body's reaction to it. Typical varieties comprise respiratory allergies, such as hay fever (allergic rhinitis) brought on by dust mites, pollen, or pet dander. On the other hand, responses to particular proteins in particular meals might result from food allergies. As an illustration, consider allergies to dairy, shellfish, or peanuts.

Direct skin contact with allergens such as specific metals, plants, or chemicals can cause skin allergies, such as contact dermatitis.

Furthermore, drug allergies may develop in reaction to drugs, whereas insect sting allergies are brought on by the venom of wasp or bee stings. Allergies may also cause conjunctivitis in the eyes as a result of exposure to allergens such as pollen or pet dander. To properly manage and comprehend the wide spectrum of allergies, one must be aware of these immunological reactions.

HOW INTOLERANCES GROW

Allergies arise from a complicated interaction between environmental and genetic variables. Allergy reactions are more likely to occur in people with a family history of allergies. The chance of developing allergies later in life might also be influenced by early allergen exposure. Specific antibodies, such as immunoglobulin E (IgE), are produced by the immune system in reaction to allergens. The body may not react to an allergen on its first exposure, but repeated exposure can cause sensitization—a condition in which the body becomes overly sensitive to the allergen—which can cause allergic reactions.

In addition, environmental variables including pollution and lifestyle modifications may be a factor in the rising incidence of allergies. According to the hygiene hypothesis, fewer viruses and bacteria may be present in early life, which could cause the immune system to overreact to harmless things and ultimately cause allergies. It is essential to comprehend the fundamental processes that lead to the development of allergies to put preventive measures and focused treatment plans into action.

RECOGNIZING ALLERGIC RESPONSES

It's critical to identify allergic reactions to monitor and intervene quickly. Depending on the type of allergen and the sensitivity level of the individual, allergic symptoms can vary greatly. Sneezing, nasal congestion, coughing, and dyspnea are examples of respiratory symptoms. Skin responses frequently show up as eczema, redness, or hives. Allergens that are consumed might cause symptoms in the digestive tract, such as nausea, vomiting, or diarrhea. Anaphylaxis, a severe allergic reaction, can cause life-threatening symptoms such as a drop in blood pressure, breathing difficulties, and throat swelling.

Diagnostic methods that assist in identifying allergens-causing reactions include skin prick testing and blood tests that measure certain antibodies. Keeping a thorough journal of symptoms and possible triggers can help identify the cause of allergies. Seeking advice from medical specialists, including allergists, is crucial for precise diagnosis and customized treatment regimens. The quality of life that an individual experiences due to allergies can be greatly affected, thus early identification and efficient care are essential to reducing the effects of allergic reactions.

COMPARING ALLERGIES AND FOOD SENSITIVITIES

Allergies and food sensitivities are both immune system reactions to specific chemicals, although they range in severity and mode of action. Known sometimes as intolerances, food sensitivities typically affect the digestive tract and are typified by difficulties breaking down particular meals. This may be the consequence of enzyme shortages, such as lactose intolerance, in which the body is unable to break down the sugar lactose, which is present in milk and dairy products. Food sensitivities, in contrast to allergies, usually do not trigger the immune system's acute reaction.

Conversely, allergies are the body's immunological response to certain foods' proteins. Histamine and other compounds are released when the immune system misinterprets these proteins and believes they are dangerous. This immunological reaction can result in a variety of symptoms, ranging from minor to serious, and in certain situations, it may even be fatal. Nuts, shellfish, eggs, and dairy products are common sources of food allergies. Allergies frequently cause symptoms including swelling, hives, trouble breathing, or, in severe situations, anaphylaxis.

THE DISTINCTIONS BETWEEN ALLERGIES AND SENSITIVITY

The length of time it takes for symptoms to manifest is a crucial distinction between sensitivities and allergies. Since sensitivity reactions can have a delayed beginning, identifying the precise trigger can be difficult. Allergies, on the other hand, usually appear shortly after an allergen is exposed. The immune system's role is another distinction: whereas sensitivities are typically associated with the digestive tract or other non-immune reactions, allergies arise from an overreaction of the immune system.

Another distinguishing feature is the intensity of the symptoms. Bloating, gas, and digestive problems are examples of milder discomforts that are typically caused by food allergies. Conversely, allergies can cause more serious symptoms, such as skin rashes, breathing problems, and potentially fatal anaphylaxis. There are differences in the testing procedures as well. For example, blood tests measuring specific antibodies can be used to diagnose allergies, while elimination diets or food diaries are sometimes needed to find triggers for sensitivities.

IDENTIFYING THE SIGNS OF SENSITIVITY

It's critical to identify sensitivity symptoms to manage and treat possible health problems. These symptoms can vary greatly and include constipation, diarrhea, bloating, gas, and stomach discomfort, among other digestive issues. Fatigue, joint pain, and headaches are some typical warning signs. Allergies to certain foods may also be related to skin conditions like acne or eczema.

It is crucial to remember that indications of sensitivity might be subtle and not always obvious right away. Patterns and possible causes can be found by keeping a food journal and recording symptoms. It is best to consult a healthcare provider for an accurate diagnosis and course of treatment. In addition, people who experience severe or ongoing symptoms can think about seeing an immunologist or allergist to rule out allergies and get the right tests for sensitivities. People are better equipped to make decisions regarding their nutrition and general health when they are aware of the differences between sensitivities and allergies.

CHAPTER THREE

CREATING THE BASIS OF A HYPOALLERGENIC DIET

EVALUATING INDIVIDUAL ALLERGIES

Establishing the groundwork for a hypoallergenic diet requires first recognizing and treating one's sensitivities. Since everyone has a different set of allergies, it's critical to pinpoint the precise triggers that could result in negative reactions?

This entails introspection as well as tracking physiological reactions to various diets. Allergies frequently cause skin rashes, intestinal troubles, respiratory disorders, and other symptoms. Understanding these expressions is essential to designing a diet that enhances general health.

ASTHMA TESTING

Although firsthand observations yield important information, official allergy testing is a more methodical way to pinpoint particular allergens. Several allergy tests, including blood and skin prick tests, can identify allergens that are difficult to identify by direct observation. These tests help create a more accurate and successful hypoallergenic diet by offering a thorough assessment of potential triggers.

Speaking with an allergist or other medical expert can help people understand the testing procedure and evaluate the data so they can make well-informed decisions.

KEEPING A NUTRITION DIARY

Keeping a thorough food record is a useful tool for monitoring eating patterns and locating possible allergies. Everyday meals, snacks, and drinks should be recorded in this notebook, as well as any related responses or symptoms.

Measuring not just the kinds of food eaten but also the methods of preparation and ingredient lists might yield useful information. Patterns may show up over time, revealing connections between particular foods and allergy reactions. This procedure encourages a proactive and knowledgeable approach to controlling food preferences.

People can also include environmental conditions, stress levels, and physical activity in the food log, as these things can affect allergic reactions. The thoroughness of this record-keeping facilitates the creation of measures to reduce exposure to allergens and provides for a comprehensive understanding of individual triggers.

Reviewing the food record regularly with medical specialists or dietitians can help fine-tune dietary modifications and guarantee continued assistance with allergy management.

Conclusively, establishing the groundwork for a hypoallergenic diet necessitates a comprehensive strategy that integrates individual consciousness, official allergy testing, and meticulous documentation.

Analyzing one's allergies prepares one for making well-informed decisions, and allergy testing offers a methodical approach to pinpointing certain triggers.

Maintaining an extensive food diary enhances these endeavors by offering current documentation of eating patterns and related responses. This all-encompassing strategy encourages a lifestyle that supports optimum health and well-being by enabling people to make decisions that are well-informed and tailored to their own needs.

CHAPTER FOUR

HOW TO MAKE A HYPOALLERGENIC DIET PLAN

NUTRITIONAL EQUILIBRIUM IN A HYPOALLERGENIC DIET

Maintaining general health and well-being while avoiding allergens that could cause negative reactions in sensitive people requires balancing nutrients in a hypoallergenic diet. The goal of a well-rounded meal plan is to satisfy necessary dietary needs by including a range of nutrient-dense foods. Achieving a balanced nutritional profile can be facilitated by emphasizing a wide variety of fruits, vegetables, lean meats, and whole grains. It's crucial to take into account alternate sources of nutrients in case allergen restrictions limit your intake.

PROVIDING SUFFICIENT NUTRITION

A hypoallergenic meal plan must pay close attention to micronutrients that may be lost when specific allergic foods are removed to ensure proper nutrition. For instance, those who shun dairy products would need to look for different ways to get their recommended amounts of calcium and vitamin D to maintain healthy bones. For assistance in creating a meal plan that satisfies specific nutritional requirements and solves any potential inadequacies related to allergen avoidance, speaking with a qualified dietitian or nutritionist might be helpful.

REPLACE ALLERGENIC FOOD INGREDIENTS WITH ALTERNATIVES

A tasty and nutritionally sound hypoallergenic meal plan is mostly dependent on the substitution of products. Finding acceptable substitutes for often allergic foods is crucial to keeping meals palatable. For example, those who are allergic to almonds can use rice or coconut flour in place of almond flour in baking recipes. Furthermore, plant-based milk substitutes for cow's milk can be used, such as soy, almond, or oat milk. Trying out different allergy-free foods not only expands one's cooking skills but also makes sure that vital nutrients aren't lost in the process.

To achieve a balanced nutritional profile, a hypoallergenic meal plan must include a wide variety of nutrient-dense foods. This strategy lessens the possibility of nutritional shortages brought on by avoiding specific allergic foods. Lean meats, whole grains, fruits, and vegetables can all supply vital vitamins, minerals, and other micronutrients needed for good health.

A careful analysis of the possible shortages resulting from the elimination of particular allergens is necessary to ensure adequate nutrition in a hypoallergenic diet. For example, those who avoid gluten might look at other high-fiber options, including quinoa or gluten-free oats. A meal plan can be customized to each person's needs by speaking with a qualified dietitian or healthcare expert. This will assist in filling in any nutritional gaps and support optimum health.

Using alternative ingredients is essential when creating a tasty hypoallergenic meal plan. Finding acceptable substitutes for items that cause allergies enables the preparation of tasty meals without sacrificing nutritious content. For example, people who are allergic to nuts can substitute sunflower or pumpkin seeds in recipes. Trying out different allergen-free components not only makes meals more varied but also guarantees that important nutrients are not missed.

A well-thought-out hypoallergenic meal plan should place a high priority on nutrient balance, delivering sufficient nutrition, and using appropriate alternative items. People can handle specific dietary limitations and maintain a fulfilling and healthful diet by adopting a wide variety of allergen-free foods.

CHAPTER FIVE

EXAMPLE MENUS FOR HYPOALLERGENIC FOODS

BREAKFAST CONCEPTS

Making a healthy and allergy-friendly breakfast is a crucial first step in creating a sample hypoallergenic food plan. It's important to choose whole foods that are simple to digest and unlikely to cause allergic reactions. Think about including different grains, like rice or quinoa, as most people with dietary sensitivity can tolerate them well. Another great option is gluten-free oats used to make oatmeal. To add a natural sweetness without using processed sugars, combine these grains with fresh fruits like bananas or berries.

Incorporating hypoallergenic protein sources like eggs, which are high in vital amino acids, should also be taken into consideration. As an alternative, you can use hemp or chia seeds for people who are allergic to eggs. Smoothies that combine hypoallergenic fruits and veggies with nondairy milk, including almond or coconut milk, make a hydrating and wholesome breakfast choice.

OPTIONS FOR LUNCH

A hypoallergenic meal plan should center lunch around a well-balanced selection of healthy fats, lean meats, and a range of veggies. Well-tolerated proteins like grilled chicken or turkey can be the star of salads or wraps. Make use of vinegar and olive oil dressings that are suitable for all allergies; stay away from typical allergens such as dairy and soy.

If you're vegetarian or vegan, think about plant-based proteins like beans or tofu. Rice bowls or quinoa topped with a rainbow of roasted vegetables make a filling and allergy-aware lunch choice. Nuts and avocados are good sources of healthy fats that enhance flavor and nutritional content.

RECIPES FOR DINNER

A hypoallergenic meal plan's dinner should be varied, tasty, and accommodating to different dietary needs. Fish that has been baked or grilled, such as cod or salmon, is high in omega-3 fatty acids and generally well-tolerated. A well-rounded and allergy-friendly supper can be ensured by serving it with quinoa pilaf or a side of steaming veggies.

Using substitute grains, such as buckwheat or millet, in place of traditional wheat goods can be a gratifying option for gluten-sensitive people. A tasty and adaptable supper option is stir-fried with an assortment of vibrant veggies and a hypoallergenic sauce—possibly made with coconut aminos rather than soy sauce.

SNACKING IDEAS

A hypoallergenic meal plan should include both healthy and handy snacks. A handful of berries or apple slices with almond butter provide a pleasant and filling snack that is free of common allergies. Crunchy and allergy-friendly rice cakes with hummus or avocado on top make a great swap for common snack foods.

If acceptable, nuts and seeds can be portioned into small portions for a boost in protein and nutrients. Personal-made trail mix, devoid of allergens such as gluten and peanuts, can serve as a flexible and highly nutritious snack choice. Furthermore, yogurt mixed with nondairy milk substitutes like coconut or almond milk combined with gluten-free granola is a tasty and filling snack that can accommodate a variety of dietary requirements.

CHAPTER SIX

HOW TO SHOP FOR HYPOALLERGENIC GROCERIES

EFFECTIVE LABEL READING

The first step in finding hypoallergenic products in the grocery store is learning how to properly read food labels. It's critical to realize that the main source of knowledge about the contents of a product is the label on food items. Seek labels that are thorough, easy to read, and include a list of all components and possible allergies. Accurately interpreting labels requires familiarity with common allergies and their alternate names. Terms like gluten, dairy, soy, nuts, and other common allergies should be closely observed. It's important to read ingredient lists carefully because some products may include derivatives that could cause allergies.

COMPREHENDING NUTRITION LABELS

Understanding the different ingredients listed on food labels is crucial to being an expert at hypoallergenic grocery shopping. Usually, ingredients are listed with the main ingredient first and in decreasing order of quantity. The allergen statement needs to specify any allergies that are present. The warnings "may contain" and "processed in a facility that also processes" should also be taken seriously since they may point to possible cross-contamination. Assistive signs like "gluten-free" or "allergen-free" certification labels are available; nevertheless, make sure to confirm which allergies they address.

COVERT ALLERGENS

For people with allergies, hidden allergens present a serious difficulty. Certain chemicals, natural flavors, and modified food starch are examples of ingredients that could have hidden allergies. You must learn about and become acquainted with these obscure sources. If unsure, ask the manufacturer for more information. It is possible to avoid unintentional exposure by keeping up with possible allergen sources that aren't always mentioned.

SAFE FOOD HANDLING AND PREPARATION ADVICE

Beyond the grocery store, there are other ways to ensure the safety of hypoallergenic meals. It's essential to handle and prepare food correctly. To prevent cross-contamination, always wash your hands well before handling allergen-free foods and use different cutting boards and utensils. Set aside particular kitchen tools for use when cooking without allergens to reduce the possibility of unintentional exposure. Inform family members of the value of preserving a hypoallergenic atmosphere when preparing food.

PREVENTING CROSS-CONTAMINATION

For those who have allergies, cross-contamination is a serious risk. Cross-contamination can be avoided by paying close attention to every detail when cooking and buying. In grocery stores, exercise caution when handling open food displays, shared utensils, and bulk bins. Establish a method at home to distinguish between products that contain allergens and those that don't. To reduce the chance of cross-contamination, properly clean and sterilize all surfaces and utensils and pay attention to shared cooking areas.

COOKING METHODS FOR MEALS FREE OF ALLERGENS

The last phase in the process of food shopping hypoallergenically is to become proficient in allergen-free cooking. Try experimenting with other items that meet your dietary requirements, like dairy-free milk, nut-free alternatives, and flours free of gluten. Investigate cooking techniques that bring out flavors without using common allergies. Excellent substitutes include roasting, grilling, and sautéing in oils devoid of allergens.

CHAPTER SEVEN

OVERCOMING SOCIAL SITUATIONAL OBSTACLES

ON A HYPOALLERGENIC DIET, EATING OUT

People with food allergies or sensitivities frequently face a special set of difficulties when dining out while following a hypoallergenic diet. It can be challenging to navigate restaurant menus because it calls for careful consideration of dietary constraints. Finding and selecting restaurants that have a track record of meeting special dietary requirements is a crucial tactic. Social media, restaurant websites, and online reviews can all offer insightful information on how well-equipped and eager the establishment is to accommodate a variety of dietary needs.

NOTIFYING RESTAURANTS OF DIETARY REQUIREMENTS

For a satisfying eating experience, it is essential to let establishments know about any dietary requirements. It's crucial to communicate your dietary requirements to restaurant workers assertively and clearly to make sure they understand. Telling the waitress about any special dietary restrictions or allergies will help them to let the kitchen staffs know. Furthermore, giving clear written directions or a dietary card can be a useful guide for the kitchen, lowering the possibility of cross-contamination or unintentional allergy exposure.

CHOOSING WELL-INFORMED MENU ITEMS

Knowledge of food preparation techniques and acquaintance with common allergens are key components of developing the skill of making educated menu selections. People should familiarize themselves with ingredients and cooking methods before going out to eat so they may choose wisely from the menu. It is recommended that patrons consult with the server or chef for advice on appropriate menu selections. This collaborative approach increases the likelihood of a secure and pleasurable eating experience.

HANDLING SOCIAL COERCION

It can be difficult to follow a hypoallergenic diet and deal with societal demands. People may find themselves in circumstances where they feel forced to violate their dietary restrictions due to peer pressure, cultural conventions, and the desire to fit in. In these kinds of circumstances, cultivating a strong sense of self-advocacy is essential. Disclosing your dietary requirements and stressing the value of your health in a polite yet strong manner helps ease social constraints and foster acceptance among friends, family, and dining partners.

EXPLICATING FRIENDS AND FAMILY ABOUT YOUR DIET

It takes time and honest conversation to properly explain your diet to friends and family. Cooperation and empathy can be increased by teaching close ones about the rationale behind dietary restrictions, the possible repercussions of consuming allergies, and the value of support. Having frank discussions and dispensing information about hypoallergenic diets can help create a community of support that values and comprehends each person's unique dietary preferences.

HONORING PARTICULAR OCCASIONS

It may seem difficult to celebrate holidays or birthdays while following a hypoallergenic diet, but it is very doable with careful preparation and inventive substitutions. To arrange a meal that works with the hosts or organizers of the event, it is helpful to let them know in advance about any dietary requirements. Bringing dishes free of allergens to share or recommending appropriate locations for the event will help ensure that everyone has a good and inclusive day.

Maintaining a hypoallergenic diet and conquering social barriers call for a proactive and knowledgeable strategy. People can successfully manage social situations without sacrificing their health and well-being by choosing places that are accommodating, communicating dietary preferences, making informed menu selections, and negotiating social pressures. To promote understanding and create inclusive workplaces for individuals with dietary limitations, open communication, education, and preparedness are essential.

CHAPTER EIGHT

SUSTAINING A HYPOALLERGENIC DIET AND A HEALTHY LIFESTYLE

EXERCISE AND ALLERGY-FREE LIFESTYLE

Sustaining a healthy lifestyle while adhering to a hypoallergenic diet necessitates a comprehensive strategy that extends beyond dietary decisions to encompass multiple facets of an individual's everyday regimen. Exercise is crucial for fostering general well-being, and those who follow a hypoallergenic diet can gain a great deal by including regular exercise in their daily routine. As part of a holistic approach to well-being, exercise supports improved cardiovascular health, metabolic regulation, and immune system function.

INCLUDING PHYSICAL EXERCISE

A hypoallergenic lifestyle that includes physical exercise must carefully take into account each person's unique sensitivities and allergies. It is important to choose activities that are compatible with one's physical state and any potential allergens. For people with allergies, low-impact activities like yoga, walking, or swimming might be great options because they reduce exposure to possible triggers. To maintain a healthy and allergy-free lifestyle, it is also crucial to consider environmental conditions while designing workout routines, such as outdoor allergens or irritants.

PARTICULAR IDEAS FOR SPORTSMEN

When it comes to athletes that have hypoallergenic dietary requirements, extra care needs to be taken. Because athletes frequently have higher energy and nutritional needs, a carefully thought-out hypoallergenic diet is required to suit these needs. To ensure optimal performance and recovery, it can be helpful to consult with a nutritionist or dietitian who specializes in hypoallergenic diets to create a personalized nutrition plan that addresses each person's unique needs, including those related to allergies and athletics.

EMOTIONAL AND MENTAL HEALTH

A healthy lifestyle must prioritize mental and emotional well-being, particularly for those who are adhering to dietary limitations. Observing a hypoallergenic diet might present difficulties that occasionally cause emotions of loneliness or frustration. Prioritizing mental health is essential, and can be achieved by practicing mindfulness, meditation, or relaxing hobbies. Navigating the emotional aspects of upholding a hypoallergenic lifestyle can be greatly aided by adopting a positive outlook and strengthening resilience.

MANAGING NUTRITIONAL LIMITATIONS

Dietary limitations can be quite difficult to adjust to, but it's important to do so with awareness and initiative. The nutritional journey might be more pleasurable by experimenting with recipes and looking into a range of hypoallergenic food options. Consulting with medical specialists, such as dietitians and allergists, can offer important insights into how to properly manage allergies. Additionally, making educated food choices and avoiding unintentional allergic reactions requires being knowledgeable about food labeling, cross-contamination hazards, and hidden allergens.

LOOKING FOR RESOURCES AND ASSISTANCE

People need to seek resources and support to maintain a hypoallergenic lifestyle. Establishing connections with individuals who encounter comparable food difficulties via online forums or support groups helps foster a feeling of belonging and empathy. Furthermore, keeping up with the latest breakthroughs in allergen-free products and substitute components, along with other developments in hypoallergenic living, enables people to make decisions that support their health objectives.

Sustaining a healthy lifestyle while adhering to a hypoallergenic diet necessitates a multifaceted strategy that includes mental and physical health, exercise, nutritional concerns for athletes, coping mechanisms, and getting help. People can efficiently negotiate the difficulties presented by food restrictions while promoting general health and vigor by incorporating these ideas into their daily lives.